Flab to FAB™
The Holistic Guide to Effortless Weight Loss

Vishal Morjaria

Praise for Flab to Fab™ from readers.

This is not just a how-to book to get healthy. It is a guidebook that inspires you to discover your inner self, a book with a physical presence and a spiritual soul. With every page you turn, you really can turn around your life. The art of getting fit has been elevated by many quick-fix books which demand you to make big changes. Flab to Fab™ knocks it off the pedestal and brings it down to earth. Getting fit and staying fit is effortless. Flab to Fab™ shows you how.

– Raymond Aaron, NY Times Best-Selling Author of Branding Small Business For Dummies and Double Your Income Doing What You Love

***

Vishal is a living example of what is possible if you simply put your mind to it and now he's given us his proven and simple to follow formula, in Flab to Fab™ to lose weight, create a healthy body, a healthy mind and healthy desires. After 20 years in this industry, this is finally a game changer.

– Alex McMillan, Founder Optimal Living 365, IDEA International Program Director of the Year Winner

***

Flab to Fab™ is a must have resource for anyone wishing to uncover the truth about eating and moving their body to become slim. vishal has packaged in a no-nonsense way, all the key elements you need to know and understand to lose weight, easily and effortlessly through good wholesome healthy eating and practical, easy to understand exercise. if you want to uncover the truth about fat loss then look no further than Flab to Fab™.

– Steve Jack, Bestselling author, speaker, coach

More praise for Flab to FAB™ from readers.

Losing weight and meeting goals were always a problem for me before following Flab to FAB™. The methods in the book have focussed me differently and brought the results I always wanted in an exciting and inspiring way. This is a new way of life.

– Maureen Harper (BA, BSc, Dip Ed.)

***

I've taken the Flab to FAB™ lifestyle programme with Vishal Morjaria for two years now and I have achieved dramatic improvements. I lost my first 10kg easily and, although the next 10 are proving harder, it is the lifestyle change that is most rewarding. I am happier, more positive, and more confident. I have moved from nutrition dominated by black coffee, red meat and red wine to one dominated by green tea, green vegetables and yellow fruits. I was diagnosed with prostate cancer. The knowledge and confidence I have gained during the programme, has enabled me to treat myself naturally, reducing it by half since diagnosis. I am now in the best period of my life.

– Dr David Harper, university Senior Lecturer

***

I was diagnosed with clinical depression. Among the many things I wanted to change were my physical wellbeing and state of fitness, and my relationship with food. So, I got in touch with Vish and joined his Flab to FAB™ fitness programme and I can tell you that now I've got a lot more energy than I had 5 weeks ago. I used to have palpitations when I woke up in the morning. I was not getting enough sleep and 5 weeks later, I have more energy and am thinking more positively. I've lost over 20 pounds in seven weeks.

– Donato Piccinno

About the Author

Vishal Morjaria is a life coach and fitness trainer. He advocates a holistic approach to fitness based on nutrition, physical exercise and positive thinking. He is passionate about life and the immense possibilities it presents, and equates being healthy with being happy and thinking positively.

From a young age, Vishal has always been interested in sports and physical fitness. He trained for the national league in a basketball academy when he was 17 and continues to actively play other sports. After completing his formal education, he worked in a bank for a while to raise the necessary capital to fund and start his own fitness and life coaching venture – Journey to Fitness (www.journeytofitness.co.uk). He sincerely believes that everyone has the right to lead a life that fulfils their potential and this is evident in the diverse lifestyles of the clients he has inspired. His clients range from young professionals leading busy lives to middle-aged and elderly adults with sedentary backgrounds.

Vishal currently lives in the UK but travels extensively as part of his work to help his clients as well as to expand his spiritual awareness. His journeys across Africa, Asia and Europe observing the different cultures and lifestyles have encouraged his belief that by making simple changes to your own lifestyle, it is possible to achieve powerful results.

Foreword

Dear healthy friend,

That's right. If you have picked up this book, then you have already taken your first big step towards a healthy, fruitful and highly fulfilling life.

Vishal is not someone who takes things lightly. In fact, he has this extraordinary strength to lift heavy weights and I do not mean those weights you find in gyms. He makes light work of heavyweight subjects like positive thinking and nourishment. He busts myths by crushing them underneath the simple step-by-step approach he presents in this book.

You may think that you are going to lose weight and get healthy by reading this book but, oh boy, are you in for a surprise?! Your life will be transformed. This book will sow the seeds for a lifelong passion to not only stay healthy and fit but also do the right thing.

The best time to read this book is after you've wasted an hour or more of your life in the gym. The worst time to read this book is later. Don't fritter away your life expending energy in useless pursuits. This book shows you how every moment and action of your life can contribute to create a fabulous lifestyle. Shed your flab and free the fabulous being within you.

Stay healthy my friend and great things will come to you.

Sincerely,

Raymond Aaron

NY Times Best-Selling Author

www.ultimateauthorbootcamp.com

The author of many bestselling books including *Branding Small Business For Dummies* and *Double Your Income Doing What You Love*, Raymond Aaron is known as Canada's #1 thought leader and success coach.

Dedication

This book is dedicated to you, the reader of my book.

The knowledge that I share with you here will enable you to take control of your mind, body and lifestyle.

Using the knowledge gained from my own struggles in life, I have charted a roadmap that you can follow to overcome the challenges and conquer the fears that can prevent you from being positive, healthy and happy.

The key to achieving life-changing results is to understand, educate, empower and encourage yourself to take inspired action.

The aim of this book is to inspire you to eliminate all traces of self-doubt, to think positively and act with confidence.

How?

By working with the elements in your life which influence your mental and physical wellbeing, I will show you how you can take control of your life.

Success is defined by your ability to find your purpose in life and then overcome everything that prevents you from achieving it.

Note to readers

The information, including opinion and analysis contained herein are based on the author's personal experiences and is not engaged in rendering medical advice or professional services. The information provided herein should not be used for diagnosing or treating a health problem or disease. It is not a substitute for professional care. Readers are advised to consult a doctor for medical advice before commencing any exercise regimen or lifestyle change programme.

The author and the publisher make no warranties, either expressed or implied, concerning the accuracy, applicability, effectiveness, reliability or suitability of the contents. If you wish to apply or follow the advice or recommendations mentioned herein, you take full responsibility for your actions. The author and the publisher of this book shall in no event be held liable for any direct, indirect, incidental or other consequential damages arising directly or indirectly from any use of the information contained in this book.

All content is for information only and are not warranted for content accuracy or any other implied or explicit purpose.

CONTENTS

CONTENTS

CONTENTS

Chapter 1

Power your success mindset

Think your ideal results
into reality

Understand your mind

It all begins in your mind. Your very existence and the world that surrounds you are created by your mind. If you think something is possible, it is. If you think it is not, then it is not. You think that the world exists, that's why it does. Illusions are nothing but a temporary reality that is created by the mind.

Your mind is a metaphysical entity that is responsible for your understanding of the process of life. Your perception of life is influenced by the reality that is formed by your mind. When someone performs an action which achieves a desired result, we say that the person demonstrated an amazing "presence of mind." In other words, the person is mindful of his or her actions.

According to psychologists, your mind thinks 60,000 to 80,000 thoughts in a day. Thinking is creating a reality. How well do you know the reality that your mind is creating? Understand your mind and be aware of the way it can influence your actions.

"Reality is merely an illusion, albeit a very persistent one." Albert Einstein

Inner world versus outer world

Your inner world is created by the process of what you are doing with yourself which in turn influences your outer world.

They are related. So, if you are unhappy about something, it originates within you. It is usually the condition your body and mind are currently in. As the saying goes, a healthy mind requires a healthy body. Your mind houses your thoughts, your desires and your ambitions. It is also the instrument through which you can transform your thoughts into actions. So, if you want to change your circumstances, then you have to start with yourself.

In order to change your outer world, you need to first change your inner world. This is the starting point. First, get your house in order then you are ready to change the world.

"Be the change you want to see in this world." Mahatma Gandhi

What are thoughts?

Your thoughts are your energy seeds, vibrating with the power to create. Picture a pleasant day in your mind. The sun is shining in a clear blue sky and the ground is flowing with the abundance of nature's bounty – green grass, lush plants and tall trees with their canopied leaves providing shelter to hundreds of chirping birds. Now zoom in on a beautiful flower in full bloom and focus on this. How did the flower originate? It bloomed because of a plant, which came from a seed. The seed grew into a plant because the elements of nature, the sun, the rain and the fertile soil nurtured it.

The human body is not unlike a plant. It needs nourishment and care. Just like the seed from which originated the plant and the other external natural elements which nurtured the plant to grow healthy and bear beautiful flowers and fruits; you need to nurture positive thoughts. The quality of the seed determines the quality of the plant and its flowers and fruits. Similarly, the quality of your thoughts will define your character and the manner in which you provide nourishment and care will influence the quality of your life.

"Life is a garden. It is an opportunity. You can grow weeds. You can grow roses. It all depends on you." Osho

Creating success

In order to achieve results, you need to envision the success that you wish to create. A fashion designer envisions a beautiful dress or a suit when she is drawing a sketch. An architect sees in his mind how the building will eventually look even when he is making the blueprint. What you create in your mind is as real as what you will physically achieve and the end results are a replication of what you visualized in the first place.

So, if your desire to possess a fab body is to come true, then you need to envision yourself possessing a body that is healthy and good-looking. It is natural to be sceptical and think how imagining something can alter the reality which is otherwise. You may not believe it at first but if you learn and apply the simple techniques mentioned in this book, you will be able to create success. Do not underestimate your power to visualize success even before it happens. You have the power to influence and transform yourself, your life and your future. Creating success begins when you envision the results even before you achieve success.

"The best way to predict the future is to create it." Peter Drucker

3-step goal setting

You can transform yourself and achieve life-changing results if you want to by using the 3-step goal setting technique that I am sharing here with you. The 3-step goal setting technique is a proven method to achieve seemingly unattainable goals and overcome challenges which are considered insurmountable.

Step 1: Set your goal. Write it down. Attach a meaning to motivate & inspire you. Set a date by when you want to achieve this goal. Be realistic but also be ambitious. For example, write down, "I want to be 10 stones 5 pounds so that I can fit into my ideal clothes, feel comfortable and be confident by 29 April 2013.

Step 2: Find a picture which excites and connects you to achieving your goal. It could be a former picture of you when you were your ideal size or it could be a picture of a role model who resembles the ideal you wish to achieve.

Step 3: This is the most exciting step. Go and get an object that will prove you have achieved your goal. Get a piece of clothing that you covet, a suit or dress that is in a size which is too small for you to fit into right now but it is the ideal size that you wish to achieve. By doing this you are staking your claim to achieve the goal and stating the seriousness of your resolve and purpose.

If you would like more support to help you in this process, please refer to one of the bonus features of this section on the website www.flabtofabbook.com, where I personally demonstrate how you can achieve your goal through the power of your thinking using this process.

"Goals are dreams with deadlines." Diana Scharf

Organize and prepare

The clearer you are in your mind, the more likely it is that you will find the process to achieve your goals, your dreams and your desires. I recommend you create systems and logs. Devise a way to regularly measure your progress.

Make daily to-do lists. Systematically log your actions and compile them in a chronological manner so you can keep track of your efforts at any point in time.

Update your logs regularly. Remind yourself of the importance of your actions using the SMART method.

Specific

Measurable

Attainable

Relevant

Time-bound

Be honest and precise in keeping track and recording your progress so you can make adjustments to alter or correct any action to make it more productive and result-oriented. Please refer to the bonus features of this section for more tips on how to organize and prepare in order to efficiently and effortlessly achieve your goals.

"Obstacles are those frightful things you see when you take your eyes off your goal." Henry Ford

Find the right support

Your personality and mindset are influenced by the people you interact with on a regular basis. You are defined by the people who are around you. Their thoughts, desires and ambitions are naturally going to affect yours. So, if you are unhappy, then it is likely that you are surrounded by unhappy people at home or at work. If you need to change, then you need to change the environment around you. Just like a plant cannot grow in an unhealthy environment, your efforts to be happy and healthy will not bear fruit if you are surrounded by people with unhealthy habits and negative thoughts. They sap your energy and prevent you from achieving your goals. To be happy and healthy, you need to be around people who are happy and healthy.

You need to create a support system or environment that nurtures your desires, encourages your efforts and provides strength and guidance to achieve your goals. You can create the right kind of support system by finding a coach, a mentor or a guide who understands your goals. You can also join a group of likeminded individuals with whom you can share experiences and exchange knowledge. If you cannot find a local support system, you can seek online support by subscribing to a blog or joining a social networking site such as Facebook or Google+.

Relying on the right kind of support can be highly beneficial by holding you accountable, providing you with expert advice, enabling you to learn from the experiences of others with similar goals and desires, and finding inspiration and encouragement when you need them most. In your journey towards fitness, your fellow travellers can guide you to achieve your goals.

"Appreciate the goodness around you and surround yourself with positive people." Nadia Comaneci

Meditation and relaxation

To renew and rejuvenate your resolve to achieve your goals, you need to replenish your inner strength. Why? Absorbing the external energy from your environment and the people around you is often exhausting. Just like you need to relax after a workout to regain your stamina, it is important to focus and contemplate on your inner world. Meditation clears the cobwebs of self-doubt and confusion. It is taking time out to be with yourself, to contemplate and be aware of your goals, and the precise actions you need to practice in order to achieve them.

Meditation bestows upon your mind clarity and sense of purpose. A source of happiness, it inspires action to achieve results. It is the calm before and after the storm. It aids in contemplation before and in reflection after a flurry of activity which leaves in its wake a churning mass of internal and external energy which may prevent you from seeing things clearly. Most importantly, it lessens the impact on the body caused by stress. It is an essential practice to achieve health, vitality and a sense of overall wellbeing.

"Empty your mind — be formless, shapeless like water." Bruce Lee

Master versus slave

You are the master of your mind not the slave. Don't allow negative thoughts to influence your mindset. Instead, control your thoughts so that you develop a positive outlook. Most people behave as if they are victims of circumstances expressing their helplessness in the way actions or situations beyond their control affect them. Instead of unnecessarily worrying about and blaming the things you cannot control, you should focus on the things you can control. The only thing you can control is your mind and your actions. This means becoming aware of your own thoughts and being mindful of your actions. Thinking positive and happy thoughts marks the beginning of taking effective and inspired action to achieve your goals.

Motivation gets you started, habits keep you going. Therefore you need to regularly practice actions required to achieve your goals. The more you apply what you have learnt, the better you will become at gaining control over your life and demonstrating that you are the master of your destiny. Do not limit yourself to a narrow mindset which prevents you from imbibing and nourishing fresh thoughts and ideas. If there is anything more dangerous than a negative mindset, it is one that is stagnant with the dogma of preconceived notions and beliefs. Set your mind free of the slave mentality and embrace the dynamic nature of positive thinking. By doing so, you will possess the power to change your destiny and the opportunity to power your success mindset to achieve the ideal results and reality you desire through your thinking.

"Your mind is your instrument. Learn to be its master and not its slave."
Remez Sasson

Conditioning

Conditioning is the collective influence that external and internal factors such as people, external experiences and your own thoughts have on your life. It is the learning that you have acquired from your experiences. When a baby is born, the mind and body are a clean slate devoid of any knowledge or awareness of what is right and what is wrong. As the baby grows up, the mind and body start responding to external stimulants and develop feelings or emotions such as love, joy, anger and fear. The environment in which the baby grows up conditions the body and mind to respond in different ways to different experiences.

So, your character and personality are a result of your experiences. You learn to react to the external stimuli based on the knowledge and awareness that you have gained. For example, as a baby, if you climbed inside an open box and felt trapped, then the memory of that incident remains within your subconscious and you exercise caution whenever you see anything that resembles a box. When you grow up this can remain embedded in your subconscious and develop into claustrophobia or an irrational fear of close spaces. Negative experiences can have adverse effects on your personality while positive experiences on the other hand can be highly motivating. It is therefore important to identify the negative experiences which are holding you back from realising your full potential. By regularly practicing and applying healthy habits and routines, you can condition your mind and body to be happy and healthy. We are creatures of habit and our habits have the power to inspire and motivate our dreams and ambitions.

"First we form habits, then they form us. Conquer your bad habits or they will conquer you." Rob Gilbert.

Positive thoughts versus negative thoughts

Your mind is a house and the thoughts that inhabit your mind can define whether it is a happy place to be or a dull and dreary place to stay away from.

Visualize positive thoughts as open windows that let in sunshine and fresh air and fill the mind with a pleasant air of joyfulness.

Negative thoughts on the other hand are like dampness and stale air that lie stagnant in a dark and gloomy house where the doors are closed, the window shutters are down and the drapes are drawn. One is a welcoming place while the other makes one feel repulsed.

Meditation and relaxation act like mirrors within your mind. When you contemplate, your positive thoughts are reflected and their brightness engenders powerful ideas and manifests itself in inspired action that enables you to move closer towards achieving your goals. Negative thoughts on the other hand do not aid in contemplation because they keep the mind murky and devoid of any illumination thereby preventing enlightenment or awareness. So, how do you condition your mind to process positive thoughts and eliminate negativity from your life?

Here are 7 steps with which you can effectively and radically go from a negative mindset to a positive one.

1. Attend a course
2. Apply what you have learned from the course
3. Get support from a coach or a mentor
4. Create or join a positive or inspirational group
5. Meditate and reflect daily
6. Surround yourself with positive likeminded people

7. Keep a journal or diary. It's a great place to start a gratitude list. Count your blessings. Be thankful for the gifts you have – your health, your happiness and the people who support and encourage you.

There is a profound connection between what you think and what you do. Your thoughts are an indication of what's going on in your life. Take care of your thoughts. They are the seeds you sow which will determine your actions and the fruits of your actions.

"The mind is its own place, and in itself can make a heaven of hell, a hell of heaven." John Milton

Psychology of weight loss

You may not be aware of it but your psychological state contributes to your physical state. In other words, your mental makeup or the thoughts that you harbour in your mind are responsible for the actions which aid in gaining weight. What, when and how you eat is a pattern that is influenced by the external environment and lifestyle that you have created which is a direct result of the way you think and perceive your inner world.

If you are unhappy with the way you look and feel, everything around you is congruent with exactly what you are thinking and feeling. Misery feeds on indolence and grows in much the same way as fat. Motivation is like a muscle, it exists within you. You need to work on it regularly to strengthen it but before that, you need to identify it.

If you wish to be healthy and happy then you have to visualize the objects which will make you feel that way. So, if you want to wear some nice clothes, then you have to go ahead and get them even if they do not fit you in your present condition. The clothes then become the motivation that drives your journey towards achieving an ideal and healthy body weight and size.

It is therefore important to understand what it is that you want, why you want it, where you are right now – your present state and where you want to go – your ideal state.

The more clarity you have in your mind about your current position and how far you are from your goal, the better you can plan and create a strategy that will enable you to reach your goal faster.

"Your body can stand almost anything. It's your mind you have to convince."
Vince Lombardi

Stress = cause

Stress is really the cause of all the negative things which affect our life including growing fat and gaining weight. I therefore define stress as the inability to deal with the internal and external forces of negativity which are adversely impacting or influencing your life. It's very easy to find out if you are stressed.

Psychologists have classified stress into seven different levels but the most common among them are mental, emotional, physical and nutritional. If you are not happy, then you are most likely not your ideal weight which in turn indicates that you are withholding stress within your body.

Look around your belly and if you are storing an excess layer of fat it is a sure indicator that there is a high level of cortisol which is a hormone produced by the body in response to stressful situations. Cortisol flows within your system and is basically responsible for storing fat around the middle of your body. As you may be well aware, fat deposited in your abdomen or belly is not only the most dangerous but also the most persistent. So attacking the symptom is futile. Instead attack the cause.

Get rid of stress.

The best way to get rid of stress in your life is to figure out what it is that you can control and what it is that you cannot. You should have realized that it is not possible to control people or situations. Attempting to do so is like banging your head against a wall. You are not only wasting your time but hurting yourself as well.

Stress tends to manifest in creating disease in your body. The key to combat stress is in your mind. Focus on taking care of your inner world and changing yourself rather than anything or anyone else. The best way to train your mind to focus is to meditate and relax as previously mentioned in this chapter. It simply means spending some quality time with yourself.

"Worry is like a rocking chair. It gives you something to do but never gets you anywhere." Erma Bombeck

Psychosomatic condition

Psychosomatic studies are concerned with the relationship between mental aspects such as stress and physical illnesses and conditions. While more and more research is being conducted in this area, it is important to understand that studies have established that there is a definite connection between your mental state and physical symptoms. In other words, your mindset and thoughts can have an impact on how your body is processing the food you consume.

It can therefore be derived that your body is but a reflection of the mental image you have of it within yourself.

So, if you are constantly having good thoughts, feeling happy and healthy emotions like love and joy, it shows in your body. It feels light, glows with vitality and absorbs good energy and repels bad energy. It is strong and is therefore better fortified from within to withstand external forces like germs and toxins which may cause diseases. If you are having thoughts which don't make you feel good, such as anger, fear or hatred, then you are very likely carrying the seeds of illnesses and diseases. Your body is therefore susceptible to even the slightest of external stimuli. When there is unhappiness within your mind it also affects your body and eventually leads to some kind of serious illness or unhealthy condition. By having negative thoughts, your body mirrors the sickness in your mind and becomes a practical embodiment of your thoughts. So think positive and be healthy.

"Natural forces within us are the true healers of disease." Hippocrates.

True story

This is a real life story of a client I've been working with. As a personal trainer and coach, I have the good fortune of working with clients across the country some of whom I don't see or meet physically. I am sharing with you here one such case study.

I had a client who was obviously quite unhealthy and unhappy as well. She was going through a very difficult time and facing multiple health and personal issues. I soon realized what was happening in her mind and how she had unconsciously created these barriers which were preventing her from regaining good health despite her best intentions. The barriers in her mind reflected the way in which she was leading her life. So her behaviour reflected what was going on in her mind.

I managed to finally figure out a way to overcome these barriers and realized that all she had to do was to reverse the process which had created those barriers. So, what we did was go through some mindset coaching, detoxing and cleansing the body along with cultivating good, healthy, organic eating habits while focussing on very light gentle movements in the form of exercise. In fact, there was very little movement at this point and it was amazing because she said that she never felt so good.

On achieving the desired results she said, "I lost 6 kilos in 28 days. I am feeling healthier and happier. I've dropped a dress size and I am simply amazed by the transformation. I am more productive, creative and positive in my attitude towards life. I feel more energetic and do not feel tired during the day like I used to. I never felt so good in almost 22 years since I got married."

This just goes to prove that by using your mind you really can do amazing things.

"I lost 6 kilos in 28 days." Priya Bhayani, UK Property Investor.

Chapter 2

Power your nutrition

Eat your way to
your ideal body and wellness

80% nutrition

80% of the results in your body are influenced by what you eat. This observation is based on my research and experiences working with clients. How healthy you are is determined by what you eat. So, if you want to see a healthy change in your body, then you should be paying more attention to the factors that influence 80% of your body which is eating and nutrition.

The mind is of course, the key driver of change but the next important element in your journey to fitness and wellbeing is nutrition. By choosing the right kind of healthy and nutritious food, you can develop a body which functions effectively, efficiently and productively. By supplying the necessary nutrition to your body, you generate the energy required to perform your regular everyday activities effortlessly and enjoy them as well.

Your energy is derived from the nutritional value of the food you eat. In this chapter, we look at smart and safe food choices and some simple yet effective methods to produce an amazing transformation in your body.

"Those who think they have no time for healthy eating will sooner or later have to find time for illness." Edward Stanley.

Detox and Cleanse

One of the simplest and powerful ways to cleanse your system is from the inside. This is one of the biggest secrets to lose fat and keep it off forever. Once you learn how to do this, you are in possession of invaluable knowledge to progressively improve your health and wellbeing, and acquire an amazing amount of energy to easily perform seemingly daunting tasks.

Most people go on quick-fix diets or a crash course exercise regimen to get back in to shape. The plethora of diets and schemes available is confusing. Most of these are not producing results because people keep going back to their original weight after trying them. There's always a new exercise fad or diet programme which promises instant results but these results are not only superficial but also temporary because they do not address the cause but just the symptoms.

The key to attaining good health is to find a simple, yet easily applicable solution which will change your lifestyle and thereby ensure benefits that will last a lifetime.

"The body is your temple. Keep it pure and clean for the soul to reside in." B. K. S. Iyengar

Dieting versus cleansing

When you go on a diet, what you are doing is reducing or eliminating the amount of calories you eat. Whether it is a soup diet or Atkins, Weight Watchers or Cambridge diet, the basic principle remains the same – to improve nutrition. One thing that none of the diets address is the toxins that remains in the body when the excess fat has gone. This may come as a revelation but it is true. The excess fat actually protects the body from the harmful effects of these toxins. In the absence of fat, the toxins are freely circulating in the body. Without fat to neutralise their effects, the body reacts creating renewed craving and appetite to bring back the fat. That's why the results don't last long because they are artificial. When the body regains the fat, it usually comes back in a bigger quantity than earlier.

All the disciplined eating habits and near-starvation comes to naught as the body returns to its previous unhealthy state. People go through this yo-yo effect, swinging between weight-loss and weight-gain, before and after a quick-fix diet. These short term makeovers are essentially causing more harm by putting the body and the mind through these dramatic changes. If you look at how the word diet is spelt and remove the last letter from it, you will realize that it actually spells die. This is a very pertinent way to remind yourself why dieting is not really healthy and how in the long run, it can kill you.

Compare the word cleansing, on the other hand, from which if you remove the letter, s, it spells cleaning. This is diametrically opposed to what dieting does. Unlike dieting which increases the body's susceptibility to toxins by getting rid of excess fat, cleansing removes toxins or harmful substances and prevents the formation of new toxins by eliminating certain food categories.

In my programme, I advise my clients on how to eat the right kind of nutrient-rich food along with the highest quality supplements in order to prevent the toxins from coming back in to the body. When you eliminate toxins and also strip away excess fat simultaneously, you are achieving long-term transformation. By acquiring an awareness of what you eat and why as demonstrated in the next step, you can become the doctor of your own health and wellbeing.

Your body has a natural ability to flush out toxins but years of consuming artificial and processed food containing chemicals and other contaminants has dulled it. Other environmental factors such as pollution have also contributed to a high amount of toxins in the body. To rejuvenate your body and regain its natural ability to expel toxins, you need to make a conscious effort to cleanse the body. Detoxing and cleansing is therefore a holistic solution to long-lasting health and well-being.

"The doctor of the future will no longer treat the human body with drugs but rather will cure and prevent disease with nutrition." Thomas Edison

What to eat and why

Your body is made up of millions of cells and the toxins are stored in the outer layer of the fat cells called the cell membrane. This is where all the poisonous elements and polluting chemicals present in the food we eat end up causing long-term damage to our body. So, if we need to focus on improving our health holistically, then we need to first build healthy cells which contribute to healthy tissues that connect our muscles, bone and skin which in turn are related to healthy functioning internal organs and a healthy system.

To eliminate bringing in more toxins into your body, you need to stop eating wheat and gluten based food. Why? If you feel the texture of gluten based food such as bread, rice, pasta and potatoes, you will realize that they are sticky substances. They clog up your digestive system and prevent your metabolism from functioning at its optimal level.

A common but harmful food element you need to stop is dairy products. Milk and almost all dairy products go through pasteurisation and homogenisation which involve subjecting milk and its derivatives to high temperatures in order to sterilize and remove harmful microorganisms. In this process, all the nutrients also get sterilized and what you get is nutrient-dead food.

Stop alcohol because it carries a lot of empty calories and sugar which is harmful to your system. Moreover, alcohol acts as a depressant and when you are making an effort to lose weight, a lack of will power does not help.

Avoid caffeine when you are detoxing and cleansing your body because it causes a high spike in your blood sugar level and leads to inconsistencies in energy, causing stress that leads to weight gain. Instead of the momentary energy rush of caffeine which does not last long, substitute it with organic energy-rich chlorophyll plant foods which provide consistent energy levels.

Get rid of sugar in your food because it is the most harmful substance and also the most addictive. It is as bad as cocaine and heroin if you consider its harmful effects. Jamie Oliver in a TED speech says how children consuming sugar is one of the main causes of the increasing child obesity rate worldwide. The biggest myth that most people believe is that fatty foods make them fat when the real culprit is sugar.

Processed food is a definite no. The conveniences and the fast-pace of a modern lifestyle have contributed to their popularity which is the main reason why incidences of illnesses has increased in the last 50-100 years. Processed food contains artificial additives and is not real food but artificially cultured chemicals. The so-called low-fat processed food is harmful because they contain artificial chemicals and is devoid of any nutrition. The myth of fat contributing to fat is misleading. In fact, essential fatty acids in the right amount present naturally in organic food are required for your daily nutrition. That's why they are called essential.

Red meat is difficult to digest and it does not help when you are focussing on improving your metabolism. There have been many cases where post-mortem reports indicated the presence of undigested red meat that is several years old. Some kinds of organic red meat are a good source of iron and it is your choice to put red meat back in your diet if you wish after you have completed the process of detoxing and cleansing.

Here's what you can you eat and drink during the cleansing and detoxing process. Drink purified water or bottled mineral water. A reverse osmosis filter is best because it ensures that all contaminants are removed. Avoid drinking tap water because it contains chemicals, pollutants and heavy metal poisoning such as arsenic and mercury which will contribute to the toxins in your body. Eat plenty of plant proteins, lentils, beans and leafy vegetables. Pour olive oil on your salads and cold food, and for cooking use coconut oil. Why? Olive oil loses its nutritional value when heated whereas coconut oil retains its nutrients even at high temperatures, offers immense health benefits and also makes your cooked food taste good. Eat organically sourced raw fruits and vegetables. These are a great source of fibre that aids in the digestive process. Also consume food rich in alkaline content as they increase the body's resistance and prevent diseases and ill health.

"If we are not willing to settle for junk living, we certainly shouldn't settle for junk food." Sally Edwards

Calories and nutrition

One of the great maladies of the modern day lifestyle is not only our eating habits but also the kind of food that is readily available. What you eat usually contains more calories and less nutrition. Therefore when we reduce calories to lose weight, the nutritional value of our food is also drastically reduced. So a person who loses weight also loses energy. This is a very unhealthy situation which promotes susceptibility to sickness due to an unhealthy and dysfunctional body.

The reason why processed food or convenience food tastes good is because, in order to substitute for their lack of nutrients, they are supplemented with additives and chemicals as well as sugar to improve their taste. Prolonged consumption of processed food conditions your taste-buds, creating an acquired taste and producing a sense of instant gratification in the body but what you don't realize is that in terms of nutritional value it is no better than eating a box of cardboard.

The hunger ratio is another damaging effect that food with no nutrients has on our bodies. When you eat natural nutrient-rich food, your stomach recognises its value for your body and sends a signal to your brain when you have consumed enough. Nutrition-less food on the other hand does not satisfy your hunger and therefore you consume more and more because your stomach fails to recognize you are overeating.

In other words, calories do not satisfy hunger. Nutrition does. Lack of nutrition in your food is the main cause of illnesses, imbalances and hormonal irregularities which lead to unhealthy, overweight and unhappy bodies.

"The food you eat can be either the safest and most powerful form of medicine or the slowest form of poison." Anne Wigmore

Organic versus ordinary food

The main difference between organic and ordinary food is the way it is grown and produced. Modern farming methods have increasingly focussed on producing more quantity of food at minimal costs. In the pursuit of profits, the quality and nutritional value of the food has deteriorated. This reduced nutritional value combined with the use of artificial fertilisers as well as the spraying of chemical pesticides to protect crops from damage has progressively been linked to the rise of illnesses in the last few decades.

Organically produced food essentially means they are free from harmful pesticides, artificial fertilisers and other forms of contaminants because the plants and the crops are naturally cultivated. Another significant difference is that organic food is locally grown and the produce is fresh unlike ordinary food which may be preserved using artificial ingredients so that they can be transported from the place they were produced to the place they are sold.

Consuming organic food is not only naturally nutritious and healthy; it also fortifies the body with essential natural elements to boost the immune system and reduce the likelihood of falling sick. Contrary to the belief that organic food is more expensive than ordinary food, organic food offers better value because it is locally grown and fresh. You are therefore not paying for the transportation or the preservatives used. In the long run, organic food can also prove to be a good investment by offsetting medical expenses as a result of eating nutrition-less food.

"The peculiar evil is that the less money you have, the less inclined you feel to spend it on wholesome food." George Orwell.

Eat clean to your ideal body

A machine needs a source of energy to function. It also needs regular maintenance. Take the example of a car. It needs fuel to run. The engine needs regular servicing to ensure that the fuel is used in an efficient manner. If you use impure fuel, then it can potentially harm the engine and prevent the car from functioning to its optimal capacity.

Similarly your body needs quality nutritional input to produce the energy required to perform everyday physical and mental activities. Food that is full of calories but devoid of any nutritional value influences the way your body functions – it becomes listless, lethargic and easily prone to exhaustion. When you consume clean, natural and organic food, your body recognises the nutritional value and is energised. Eating processed and artificial food is just like putting impure or adulterated fuel in a car or any machine; it will either reject the fuel or lead to malfunctioning and eventually a breakdown.

In our pursuit of creature comforts and conveniences, we have relegated taking care of our body as the least priority and our health and wellbeing has naturally been affected by the neglect. The evidence is all around us, rising illnesses, obesity, premature aging and the poor quality of life when health is not the main priority. It is not difficult to bring back healthy practices into our daily routine. Using the awareness you have gained from this book about the kind of food to eat and the reasons to do so, you can apply the knowledge to effect a life-changing transformation.

Acquiring health requires just a series of small changes that involve discipline and determination. Once you start practicing what you have learnt here, you will immediately experience physical and emotional benefits. You will take pride and joy in your body's ability to perform tasks effortlessly which previously seemed difficult. Your body becomes a vehicle of happiness. After all, if you don't take care of your body, who will?

"You don't have to cook fancy or complicated masterpieces – just good food from fresh ingredients." Julia Child

Easier and more effective than killer training

The irony is that most people who go to the gym and burn themselves out by working out would be much better off if they spent the time acquiring some basic knowledge about nutrition and use this awareness in their daily lives. Then instead of going for killer exercise regimens which are actually killing their enthusiasm and their energy, they will eat nutritious food and generate more energy to exercise.

I therefore advice you to use the knowledge you have acquired here and leverage your awareness that 80% of your body's health and wellbeing is a result of nutrition to implement a healthy and long-term lifestyle change, the benefits of which you can reap for a lifetime.

Even if your primary goal is to lose weight and achieve your ideal body size, by practicing the methods mentioned in this book, you will gain not only physical but emotional and psychological benefits as well. The result – you will be healthier, happier and mentally more active and become more positive in your attitude.

By eating healthy, you will be able to achieve the body weight you desire and deserve.

"One cannot think well, love well, and sleep well, if one has not dined well."
Virginia Woolf.

Role and importance of high quality natural organic supplements

If you eat natural, fresh and organic food, then do you really need nutritional supplements? Are nutritional supplements really beneficial or just a panacea? The controversy surrounding the use of food supplements and the value they can provide has led many of us to question their relevance and importance.

I was always a believer that you can get all the nutrients that you need from eating natural food. However, as I will explain and demonstrate in the later chapters of this book, I found from my experiences that you cannot get all the nutrients that are essential from the food that is usually available. This is mainly because of the way food is produced. Therefore I conducted a detailed research on the food supplements available in the market and tried to identify the highest quality herbal supplements that are traded and sourced fairly, ethically and with integrity. Following my research and experimentation with various supplements and brands, I finally chose Nature Sunshine and found out that they have the largest range of the highest natural quality herbal supplements that produced dramatically significant results.

I have found that people who supplemented their nutritional intake of organic food with these supplements have seen great improvements in their health.

Whenever I am involved in an important decision which concerns nutrition, I conduct a thorough investigation and aim to educate, empower and enable you to understand why you are eating what you are eating. This precedes any advice I give my clients in my programme. In my coaching, I endeavour to explain to my clients what is going on within their system and what specific steps they can take to achieve their health goals. I analyse individual health goals and customise my programme to your requirements accordingly. Compare the personal analysis of your individual requirements to the MOT test you would conduct for your car. As a gift from me to you, I am going to give you the opportunity to do a personal analysis absolutely free of charge when you sign up at www.flabtofabbook.com

"About 80% of the food on shelves of supermarkets today didn't exist 100 years ago." Larry McCleary

Chapter 3

Power your body

Move your body to
your ideal body shape

20% exercise

Now that you know that 80% of the results in your body come from nutrition, combined with 20% results from physical exercise, you can apply this knowledge and put it into practice to achieve the transformational results you desire from your body. It's important to understand how exercise affects your body to effectively use it to your advantage.

Exercise acts as a catalyst and one of its functions is to speed up the metabolism process within your body which helps to burn fat. You may recall a science experiment that you did in school, where you took a small strip of magnesium and burnt it. What this experiment demonstrates is that though magnesium on its own is combustible or has the potential to burn, it cannot do so without a catalyst. The catalyst, in this case the flame, is required for magnesium to overcome its activation energy and burn. Similarly, exercise is a catalyst that stimulates the body's ability to burn fat. So, with the right kind of exercise complemented with the right kind of nutrition, you can get the results you desire.

"Nobody is worth more than your body." Melody Carstairs

Smart effective training

Most people train their bodies for hours performing strenuous activities and yet end up with no results. Sometimes the results are the opposite of what they desire. Their bodies end up being in worse shape than when they started, fatter and fatigued. They wonder why they are not getting the results they desire despite their best efforts. They don't realize the importance of nutrition. It is equally important to identify the right kind of training that will determine the outcome of your exercise, replacing repetitive and exhausting exercise routines with varied intervals of energetic movements.

It is definitely not the quantity of the exercises or for how long you sweat which counts. It's the quality or how you practice your movements that matters. Instead of spending hours at the gym, if you could do your workouts as effectively and efficiently in 20 to 30 minutes daily, imagine how much time you could save so that you can do other activities which you value in your life? This is one of the main reasons why 80% of gym members don't actually achieve the results they desire and end up leaving.

"Train, don't strain." Arthur Lydiard

Fat-storing versus fat-burning

Imagine turning your body from a fat-storing machine to a fat-burning machine. You can do this when you change the methodology of your training from long, boring and enduring sessions to short, enjoyable and effective efforts. By this I mean high interval resistance training which will teach your body to increase its metabolism rate in a natural way. What this means is that while you are going about your regular activities at home or at work, you can train your body to work for you rather than against you.

In other words, you condition and enable your body to consistently and regularly burn fat and convert it to energy instead of allowing your body to revert to storing fat during periods of rest. This is the secret to energize your body without spending too much physical time working out.

"If it doesn't challenge you, it doesn't change you." Fred DeVito

Do less and achieve more

You often see most people who spend a lot of time in the gym, and you may be one of them, get frustrated because they are not getting the results they think they deserve. They spend two or three hours or sometimes even four hours a day and yet at the end of it all they don't have any results to show. Why?

You are obviously doing something wrong if you are not getting results. This chapter highlights the importance of working smarter instead of harder, how you can achieve more by doing less and how you can go from poor or no results to phenomenal life-changing transformation. How?

Change what you are doing right now. It may be difficult to challenge conventional methods because our minds and bodies have been conditioned to believe that the harder and longer you work, the easier it is to achieve results. However, don't you realize that you are only making it harder and not easier? You may find it hard to do the opposite of what you have been told is good for you. It is however important that you challenge and remove the mental and physical conditioning that you have acquired in order to achieve results effortlessly.

It is possible when you have the necessary support and guidance in place. You can do this when you work with a fitness coach who will work with you to identify the right kind of exercises and by varying the intensities in an effective manner to produce optimal results. The main objective is to ensure that the effects of your workout last longer and your body reaps the benefits of the workout even while resting. By doing this, the results you desire and deserve materialize with dramatic ease.

"Movement is a medicine for creating change in a person's physical, emotional and mental states." Carol Wench

Movement and joy

Your body is designed for movement. Once you recognize this fundamental truth, then you realize how easy it is to do some of the things which you thought were practically impossible. Have you seen acrobats and gymnasts perform and watched with envy their graceful movements and how effortlessly they seem to do it? The secret lies in the joy with which they perform these activities.

Once you realize that you can also enjoy physical workouts and exercise and start practicing it regularly, you will be amazed at the variety of movements you are capable of and how you can use these to achieve your ideal body weight and image.

Going to a gym is not the most enjoyable activity. For most of us it is a chore that you have to get through than something you look forward to. Most often this is because you see going to the gym as performing boring routine movements in a closed box.

Your body is created to enjoy freedom of movement and the joy of living comes from this. Though some of us may enjoy going to the gym, most of us would rather be outdoors, breathing in the fresh air, feeling the sun on our skin and doing the kind of movements that come to us naturally and effortlessly.

It is important to discover the movements that bring you joy because then, you will want to do them more often and feel less tired. If your workouts are leaving you exhausted rather than energized, then this is a sure sign that you are not enjoying it. When you discover movements that are joyful, you are not merely exercising but living them. You are being mindful of performing them and thereby maximizing the results and enriching your body. You will develop a stronger connection and a better appreciation of your body which is the vehicle that will take you towards achieving your goals.

I want you to apply this simple method to discover the movements that bring you joy. Take a pen and paper and write down as many movements as you can that you have done and have brought you joy or movements that you wish you could do and which you think you will enjoy. Make sure that your list contains at least three items. It could be something as simple as going for a walk or something that you did when you were a child such as performing cartwheels or something that you aspire to such as yoga. Once you have made your list, put down the reasons why you think you enjoy doing them and next to that a date for each item to indicate when you will start doing them, if you are not doing them already. Presto! You are already on your way to get the maximum benefits doing the movements you enjoy.

"Number one is to gain a passion for running. To love the morning, to love the trail, to love the pace on the track, and if some kid gets really good at it, that's cool too." Pat Tyson

Modern day exercise versus olden day exercise, gym exercise versus alternative methods

It is a place filled with positive energy where you can find hopeful people working really hard to achieve targets that they are not even remotely aware of. Does this sound familiar? I must admit that it is one of the best descriptions for the gym that I've come across. The best part, they say, is that a gym is a great place to see and meet good-looking men and women. The reality, unfortunately is not so and you soon realize that there are more people trying hard and less people achieving results. Why?

Gyms are just places where there are tons of equipment and weights. It is definitely a place you can go to train but gyms don't guarantee results except profits for those who run them. On the brighter side, you don't have to go to a gym to get results. There are many alternative ways to train which are not only more effective but less costly and time-consuming. For example, you can buy some very simple functional tools and exercise kits which can be used almost anywhere, in a small space within your home, outdoors in a park or on a terrace, in your garage, where you can absolutely enjoy the freedom of doing these movements.

I have spent a good part of over 5 years working in a gym environment and realized that it was not natural and it did not feel right. I would constantly encounter people working till they get tired and moving backwards in terms of achieving their goals instead of being energized and motivated, and moving closer towards their goals. The fact is that a gym is where people go to empty their guilt of eating unhealthy food or leading an unhealthy lifestyle. It therefore starts resonating with this negative energy that people who come here leave behind by working-out to burn some calories that they hope will make them feel better for not doing the right things. This, I think, is a pathetically hopeless and half-hearted way of achieving the ideal body weight.

I believe that if you can do physical movements that you enjoy, you can achieve great results no matter where you do them. The most important thing is to identify what you enjoy and do it in such a way that you are energized and rejuvenated before, during and after. Even when you feel tired, there is a sense of achievement.

"If I were to draw on a paper what gym does for me, I would make one dot and then I would erase it." Elizabeth Berg

My sample workout

You can visit my website www.flabtofabbook.com and pick up some of the exercise programmes that are mentioned there which will guarantee you great results. While writing this book, I was recovering from a broken wrist and I have not done any training for over two months. I have not done any road running for over 3 years and I am training to take part in a half marathon with only four weeks to prepare for it.

I am telling you this because I want you to know that it doesn't matter if you have not been doing something for a long time, you can still start and achieve your goals if you have a plan. I am doing this also to prove to myself that I am up to challenging myself just the way I am pushing my clients to challenge their limits.

I am practicing what I preach.

I am also preparing myself for the basketball season in division one which means that I haven't played at a competitive level in the league for almost 6 years. This shows that I am also identifying and doing the movements that I enjoy just like I ask you to.

I usually prefer to do 20 to 30 minute workouts 3 to 5 times a week using body weights or other fitness equipment such as Kettlebells, ViPR and playing sports that I enjoy such as football or basketball. If you are a beginner, I highly recommend you start with body weights and then move onto advanced types of training.

I would always advise you to change and vary your training every 4 to 8 weeks in order to make sure that your body keeps adapting and moulding to your ideal shape.

I prefer doing workouts which help me train smarter and for a shorter time while boosting my body's metabolism so that I get optimal results. By understanding how my workouts are affecting me, I can progressively achieve better results and continue to maintain a naturally healthy weight and body shape. So can you.

"Nothing will work unless you do." Maya Angelou

Chapter 4

Power your lifestyle

Live well, fulfil your dreams, desires
and achieve greatness

Harmonise mind and body to live the dream life

Now that you are aware of the connection between the mind, nutrition, movement and the significance of their influence on your health, you can start putting them together. In order to achieve your dream life or a great lifestyle, you need to combine these three essential elements – what you think, what you eat and how you move your body. Most people miss this simple point – that a happy and healthy life is the result of an integration of these seemingly diverse elements. Through this book, you will realize the importance of adopting a holistic view of health and wellbeing. Harmonise the different elements that contribute to health and when you consciously guide them to achieve the ideal balance, health and wellness will naturally materialise in your life.

What people see on the outside is actually the result of what happens within you. You are creating the lifestyle of your dreams inside out. Remember that through your mind and your thoughts, you have the power to visualize the lifestyle you desire and deserve. By creating a clear picture in your mind of what your heart desires and consciously nourishing these desires with the right kind of nutrition and physical activity, you will be able to transform what you have visualized into reality and improve the quality of your lifestyle. What you think about, you can bring about.

"Body and mind, and spirit, all combine to make the creature, human and divine." Ella Wheeler Wilcox.

Prevention strategies

According to Charlotte Gerson of the Gerson Institute, most people don't focus on prevention but are more concerned in attending to symptoms. They only take action when there is something drastically wrong with their health. They have a very reactive relationship with health and well-being instead of being proactive and taking positive steps to safeguard their health and wellbeing. This attitude is the result of a complacent mindset that takes the body and health for granted.

It's like washing your car and making it shine from the outside but not paying attention to the fuel tank when it is empty. Your body cannot run on an empty diet that does not provide it the necessary nourishment. Just like a car with a near-empty tank is going to suffer a breakdown at any moment, a body that lacks quality natural nutrition despite being filled with processed and artificial food will give up, and that's when most people wake up and acknowledge the damage that their own actions have caused.

Imagine being able to foresee what results or outcome your actions will bring. Will you still continue practicing them if you knew that they can cause irreparable damage? Logic demands that you do not. Yet, many people turn a blind eye to the unhealthy food they eat and the lack of exercise in their lives until something terrible or life-threatening jolts them out of this complacency. I have heard clients say that they wish they knew the damage that they were causing so that they could have prevented something terrible or awful from happening. That is why I always say that it is better to prevent now than repent later.

For every effect there is a cause. By this I mean, that any outcome is the result of an action and the action was inspired by a thought. It all begins in the mind. Once you understand the cause and effect theory and apply its relevance to your life, you will recognise that you are responsible for everything that happens in your life.

They say it takes a great deal of courage to accept responsibility but if you breakdown the words that form responsibility, you get respond and ability which is basically your ability to respond to a situation. So when you find that you are unhappy with your body, circumstance or situation, instead of playing the victim and doing nothing, use your ability to respond in a positive and constructive manner. Accept the fact that your actions are responsible for the current situation. This may be the hardest thing to do but once you do so, then you will witness that your life has the potential to change positively and powerfully. Use the realisation that your actions caused the effect and with this newfound awareness and understanding, you will have the power to change the situation to your advantage. Remember you can influence what's outside and around you only by changing what's inside you.

Let me show you by using myself as an example of how I could transform my life. Let's say that I am unhappy with the way I look and feel. I realize that I have to change the way I think about myself, what I am eating and how much I am moving my body. So, I decide to go on a programme to change the way I look and feel. Initially, I will need lots of support to get started. I will need guidance and mentoring but even before all this, I need to be inspired to take the steps to start moving towards the change I desire. I can do this only by taking responsibility for my actions; that is use my ability to respond to what my mind thinks. Once I harmonize the mind and the body, then I am in control of my life and can change myself and by doing so, influence a change around me and the circumstances in my life.

Only you have the power to make a difference by taking responsibility to produce the positive outcome that you desire.

"An ounce of prevention is worth a pound of cure." Benjamin Franklin

Live with love

If you go through life with a bitter tongue, saying that you are unhappy, then your thoughts and behaviour are influenced by the bitterness. On the other hand, if you decide to have a sweet tongue and say good things, then you can be happy and you can have a better life instead of a bitter one. Learn to love unconditionally all that you come into contact with because you share this planet with others who are your companions. According to the law of giving and receiving, when you give love naturally and freely, you will receive love in return. By living with love and giving love to those around you, you are contributing to the abundance of love that exists on this planet. The more love you give, the more you will receive. This is an indisputable fact and you can experience it yourself.

Each of us is a servant of the life we live and everything you do is for the greater good of mankind and this universe. Adopting the mentality of being a servant of life and doing service to those around us requires us to be humble. When you let go of your pride, you will be able to reach out and influence the minds and hearts of the people around you. When you serve life in this way, you will witness how your life is magically transformed from being empty and meaningless, and becomes full of opportunities and possibilities.

Begin with yourself. Love and respect yourself and treat yourself the way you would treat the person you love the most in this world.

When you begin to treat yourself and serve your own life, then only will you be able to treat others with love and respect.

"Love the life you live. Live the life you love." Bob Marley

Think your way to your dream life

What is it that you really want? Why do you want it? By when do you want it? How do you plan on getting it? These are some of the most important questions that you can ask in your life. To achieve your goals, it is important to have a clear picture in your mind. When you are clear about the what and the why, the how will come to you naturally.

The most powerful and profound way of getting what you want in life is to visualize it. The more clarity you have, the easier it is to put in the necessary efforts to get closer to your goals.

Always remember that your dream life may change many times during the course of your life. It is therefore important to constantly ask yourself these questions and renew your goals and desires. Writing down your goals will enable you to find clarity in your thoughts and desires. Visualizing and bringing them to life with pictures that represent your dream life will enhance and energize your efforts to achieve them. By translating your thoughts and desires into words and pictures, you are projecting them from your mind to the external world and this is the beginning of your journey to achieve your dream life.

Contemplate your desires.

Spend some quality time with yourself; reflect in silence and solitude on your dream life and you will create inspirational thoughts and ideas to achieve them. The important thing is to think but thinking alone is not enough. You need to have inspired thoughts and inspired actions in order to make your dreams happen.

I want to share with you my own experiences to show you how you can achieve what you desire if you work on it. I recently travelled down the south coast of Spain and around Gibraltar. Not only was my trip paid for but I also got paid while on the trip, for just being myself and inspiring others. It was a lifestyle that I never dreamt could be real. It was as if I never believed that I could have created the opportunity until I realized that the dream lifestyle was a result of my own inspired thoughts and actions. Something which I felt was impossible, which I would spell as I'm possible, is now possible because of my own thoughts and actions. If it is possible for me to achieve my dreams, then it is also possible for you.

Start today by thinking and clarifying your thoughts.

"When you cease to dream you cease to live." Malcolm Forbes

Die theory and philosophy

Ask yourself, if you die today, what will die with you? Asking this question will give you a clear understanding of what dreams are currently residing within you and remain unfulfilled. It brings clarity of perception on how you see yourself.

The truth is that most people when they are going to die regret not having lived the life they dreamt of. Your life is an opportunity to realize your dreams. Don't fritter it away by allowing your fears and worries to hold you back. You can have all the greatness you wish for if you let go of negative thoughts and embrace positive thoughts.

Make a decision today that you will not be held in a prison of negativity and instead will seek the freedom of positivity. Go ahead and live the life of your dreams. There is nothing that can prevent you from achieving the greatness you desire and deserve except your own fears and doubts.

Ask yourself, what will make me realise my true potential? Is it doing voluntary work? Is it trying to be a better father or mother? Is it taking better care of my health? Is it achieving financial stability? Is it travelling and seeing the world? Treat today as the day you would die and do the things you always wanted to do. Ask yourself, if I die will my dreams die with me and will I leave behind regrets? Or will you leave behind a legacy that will inspire others to follow their own dreams?

"If you live each day as if it was your last, someday you'll most certainly be right." Steve Jobs

People

People are a big part of life. Their presence forms a huge influence in how you live your life. The quality of the people who are around you will not only determine the quality of your life but also define who you are. The company you keep colours your character. If you are surrounded by positive people, you will be a positive person. If not, then your life is a recipe for disaster because negative people will prevent you from achieving what you want, even if you try very hard.

How to identify negative people? They are the ones who will keep telling you that you cannot do this and that because they are afraid to realize their own dreams themselves. They will therefore discourage you from living the life you dream of because they themselves are not. If you are not careful, being surrounded by negative people will influence you to think like them. Their negativity is infectious and will affect your life just like a virus and without realizing it, you will start having fears, worries and doubts about your own life where none existed before.

It is in your best interests to stay away from negative people because they are not interested in your success but they are jealous and envious that you may succeed where they didn't.

On the other hand, with positive people around you, you will feel energized by their own dreams and desires and they will also encourage you to pursue your own dreams as they are doing. Their enthusiasm will keep you going. The choice to be with the right kind of people is yours and forms an important part of your journey towards achieving your dream lifestyle.

I always make a conscious effort to associate and connect with positive people who wish to make this world a better place and I highly recommend that you do so too.

"Positive things happen to positive people." Sarah Beeny

Chapter 5

It's powered by lies

What modern day health and food
industries don't share, educate or teach

Cycles of control

In this chapter, I will show you why it is important for you to take control of how you live your life because if you do not there are other forces at work which will.

The whole global economic system is influenced by a few major international corporations and companies. Their influence extends to your personal choices and decisions through the advertising messages that you receive on a daily basis. Unless you become more conscious of the way you think and are also more aware of how these companies operate, you will continue doing just what these companies want you to do so that they can make more profits while your health and wellbeing is being adversely affected by your actions.

Companies such as Monsanto for example, create chemicals which are used to genetically modify and produce food which is then sprayed with pesticides and fungicides to protect the food crop from being damaged. This food is then injected or treated with even more chemicals to preserve it so that it will have a longer shelf life and look attractive. Their main argument for doing this is that it is required in order to meet the growing demand for food caused by the ever-increasing world population. However, I believe there surely are better ways to maximise resources and improve productivity without sacrificing the health and wellbeing of consumers. The fact remains that for these companies, the interest of the consumer is secondary compared to the imperative to make profits.

The food that we buy in supermarkets around the world, whether it is 'fresh' fruits or vegetable, is transported over long distances and is therefore not really 'fresh' but preserved using artificial preservatives. So when we consume these food items which are genetically modified, we are inadvertently consuming unnatural chemical substances which weaken our immune system and cause illnesses. When we are ill, we see a doctor who prescribes medicines to treat the symptoms rather than the real illness. Believe it or not, the pharmaceutical companies that manufacture the medicines are connected to the companies that produced the genetically modified food and the chemical preservatives that made you ill.

So, the chemicals in the food that we eat which is responsible for the sickness that the doctor treats using medicines that are all produced by the same corporations – they are all part of a vicious cycle of control. The saddest part is that the medicines are only providing temporary relief because they are addressing only the symptoms but not the seed or the germ which is due to lack of nutrition in the food that we eat. Doctors are doing the best they can but if you take into account the fact that nutrition occupies just 3 to 5 hours duration in their 5 to 7 years of medical training, you will realize that the most effective means of ensuring good health is in your hands.

You need to empower yourself with the knowledge and awareness of what is good for your health and focus on the nutritional needs of your body in order to take control of your health and wellbeing.

"He who cannot obey himself will be commanded. That is the nature of living creatures." Nietzsche

Nutritional deficiency and toxic overload

As demonstrated in the earlier part of this chapter, modern day farming practices are focussed more on the quantity of the produce as opposed to quality. The demands of mass production have also led to agricultural practices that are adversely affecting the quality of the soil. As more and more crops are harvested round the year, the natural ability of the soil to replenish itself is diminished and this in turn affects the quality of the crops that are produced in the soil. Because of being highly overused, the same soil that produced nutritious food grains, fruits and vegetables before are now unable to produce the same quality of food. That's why the nutrients which were naturally present in our food 50 to 100 years ago is no longer available. This is why it is essential to fortify your nutritional intake with high-quality organic nutritional supplements. Please visit www.flabtofabbook.com which provides relevant information and resources on the highest quality herbal, vitamin, mineral and nutritional supplements.

While the food we eat has been diminishing in nutritional value, all kinds of pollution in the air, soil and water is contributing to a growing toxic presence in the elements around us. We are constantly being exposed to harmful toxins in the air we breathe, in the food we eat, the clothes we wear and in many other ways when we come in contact with the environment. Simple sources of sustenance such as the tap water we drink is contaminated by pollutants and toxins which are slowly but surely degrading our health and wellbeing.

The presence of the toxins is responsible for damaged and dysfunctional cells and their effects gradually permeate from the cells into our system and organs unless we check their progress and take precautionary measures. That is why I highly recommend you to go on a detox and cleansing protocol as detailed on my website www.flabtofabbook.com

"Expect poison from the standing water." William Blake

Your mind is suppressed through social control

This may sound like a conspiracy theory at first but what I am sharing with you here is what I believe to be true and is a result of my research and first-hand experiences. Most people have been distracted by multiple media interactions such as television, music, radio, computers, mobile phones and the internet. The barrage of influences that these external elements are having on us is indescribable. We often see people wearing earphones while walking or exercising, or sitting for hours glued to the computer or the TV. They are literally plugged into one of these external media all throughout their active lives.

The truth is that most people are afraid to think or contemplate on their own. They therefore unconsciously yet deliberately and willingly distract themselves and ignore what is really going on in their minds. They seek superficial distractions so as not to face reality or develop a deeper understanding of their awareness.

There are innumerable ways in which your mind is being conditioned without you being aware. You may be seeing different images on TV which influence your mind to think that a certain body shape or look is what is healthy and ideal when you are not even questioning the reality of the suggestion. When you see a certain body shape as being undesirable and it coincidentally reminds you of your own body, you are unconsciously causing yourself to have low self-esteem.

The primary intention of advertising and marketing is to make profits for the manufacturers of the products and not to enhance your health or wellbeing. That is why it is important to cultivate clarity in your mind about what it is that you really want.

Detach yourself from external influences once in a while and plug into your inner awareness.

Meditate, contemplate and spend quality time with yourself instead of being constantly distracted by social interactions with the external world.

"Laws control the lesser man. Right conduct controls the greater one." Mark Twain

Become your own doctor

You know that doctors can be relied upon to treat the symptoms of sickness. But do they actually heal your body and prevent illnesses? Do they address the core issue of what really causes illnesses in the first place?

The way to prevent illnesses is to take control of your life and take the necessary precautions. You can be the doctor of your own health and wellbeing by using the knowledge and awareness that you have gained from this book to power your nutrition by eating the right kind of food and by powering your body with the movements that you enjoy in combination with adopting and cultivating a positive and healthy mindset. This way you are not just curing the symptoms but holistically healing your body from the inside out and also transforming your lifestyle by achieving life-changing results.

You have the choice of living a life that is dependent on external forces or make the transition to take over the controls and steer your life consciously towards your goals. Instead of passing on the responsibility of taking care of your health to others who may not have the appropriate ability to respond to your needs, you are in much safer hands when you control what happens in your life by focussing on prevention and the cause rather than the symptoms and effects.

You can grope and stumble in the darkness that external elements are creating through their continual influence in your life or you can achieve the freedom that is bestowed upon those who seek enlightenment through their own efforts to understand and empower your awareness.

"Your beliefs can be your medicine or your poison." Steve Maraboli.

Change your life and influence your family

You know that you cannot change others or the situation around you but you have the power to change yourself.

When you align yourself with your newfound purpose and passion to effect a positive change from within, you will be able to inspire the people around you to emulate your example. By changing yourself, you are proving to those around you that it is possible to achieve your goals by empowering yourself.

You are setting in motion a chain of influence that will spread and embrace not only people but the circumstances that surround your life. You become a source of positive influences and it will be reflected in your surroundings. Your immediate family and friends with whom you interact will begin to notice the change in you, and you become a living example of the transformational results that is possible for everyone who wants to change for the better.

Not only will you make your nearest and dearest family and friends proud of your achievements but your transformation will speak for itself and convince even those who lacked confidence in you or doubted your abilities to respond and take control of your life.

"Things do not change. We change." Henry David Thoreau

You can be the difference

All change begins with you. There exists within you a bright light and energy that you may not be aware of until you activate it. It is like a dormant powerhouse that has the potential to inspire change within you and through your actions help and enrich the lives of millions of people. Do not underestimate your own powers to effect a change. You are an important part of the great universe we live in and the greatness that you can potentially contribute can be realized only through your thoughts and actions. So focus on consistently developing, growing and expanding your awareness, and by achieving your goals, you will make a difference and make this world a better place.

"Everybody thinks of changing humanity but nobody thinks of changing himself." Leo Tolstoy

Chapter 6

Power your actions

How to take inspired action
to get results?

What is inspired action?

Before you do something significant or important, there is usually a deliberate thought or idea in your mind which propels you to take action. We are not talking about routine things that you do as part of your everyday life like getting out of bed or brushing your teeth or tying your shoelaces. What we mean is the kind of action which sometimes you are afraid of doing but do anyways, the kind of action which you have never done before or which you may have done a million times but have never done it with the kind of mindfulness that you are going to do now or in the future.

It could be something remarkable such as when an athlete takes part in a race because he feels that it is his destiny to run and win. It could also be something as simple as replying to an e-mail with sincerity.

Inspired action begins within you, with a willingness to create or do something which you know will make you feel good. This is the kind of action that is born in moments that you spend in silence, pondering and reflecting upon your inner desires and goals.

Isn't it better to do something you really want than just do something?

Inspired action begins in your mind, with a thought or an inspiration and it remains unresolved until you act upon it. The inspiration is so strong that all objections or unwillingness that you may have in performing the action breaks down in its presence and this is where greatness is born.

You may be putting off doing something by making excuses and saying that you are not ready. You may mistake this for perfectionism but there is a fine line between procrastination and perfection and I will show you why it is important to seize the moment when you have an inspiration and do it. Once you learn to trust your instincts and distinguish between impulsive action and inspired action, you will begin your journey towards achieving your goals.

"You don't have to be great to get started, but you have to start to be great."
Les Brown

Why most people stop successful results from coming to them?

We are responsible for our actions and our actions are responsible for the situations that we create. Some people are afraid to do things that will bring them success while others say that they are not successful because they are not lucky. It is easy to justify failure but it is not always easy to live with the realisation that you could have had the success you wanted, if only you had acted upon your thoughts and desires. Here are the three reasons why people willingly prevent successful results.

1. Procrastination.

It is the worst enemy of inspired action. People often procrastinate or delay doing things they don't enjoy or avoid doing things which they feel they are not good at. These feelings come from finding out that these actions either do not fulfil them or they find it a waste of time and would feel better doing something else instead. The way to overcome procrastination is to focus on doing things that you love. For example, if you love eating but do not like cooking then to prevent yourself from going hungry, you need to find support or assistance to get the cooking done by someone else

2. Excuses.

Most people spend more time and energy justifying inaction than it would really take to act and find out the truth. They don't realize that the only people who are preventing them from getting what they want are themselves. They are living in a prison of their own making, built by self-doubt and irrational fears. These are negative thoughts and the more you allow them to grow, the less likely you are going to do anything. When you hear words like but, what if, can't or shouldn't, beware. These are the product of negative thoughts. People who say they are afraid of failure are afraid of success. They create their own obstacles and barriers. To achieve success, you have to excuse your excuses.

3. Blame.

This is a sign of weakness and immaturity. Have you noticed how guilty children look when you ask them who did it? They point at each other. Have you also noticed how grown-up, they appear when they willingly step forward and accept responsibility for something they did? To avoid taking responsibility for their actions most people take the easy way out and find someone or something to blame. It's usually other people, circumstances or luck.

As Mahatma Gandhi said, "When you point your finger at someone, remember that three fingers are pointing back at you." Those who don't take responsibility are those who haven't taken control of their own lives and expect others to control and guide them so that they can blame them when they don't get what they want. But the fact remains that they are bound to fail because they are not doing what they want but what others want.

"You miss 100% of the shots you don't take." Wayne Gretzky

How to be an inspired action taker?

You have to focus on the reason you are doing something. Once you realize that why you are doing something is more important than what it is that you are doing, your action will be driven by the force of inspiration and you will tap into a newfound source of energy and enthusiasm that you have never experienced before.

To get you started on your journey towards a life filled with inspired action, I have identified five key elements which will enable you to tap into your inner strength.

1. Find a coach or mentor to guide you and clarify your goals and desires.
2. Define your goals by writing them down and actualising your intent to achieve them.
3. Seek support from friends and family so that you can share your goals.
4. Interact with positive people in order to take inspiration and emulate their actions.
5. Join a group of likeminded people, online or on location and learn from their experiences.

Remember that the inspiration to take action comes from within you. However by positively engaging with people around you, you can create the right environment to achieve success.

"Knowing is not enough, we must apply. Willing is not enough, we must do."
Leonardo Da Vinci

Think less do more

Every action begins in the mind.

The thought is the seed; the action is the plant that grows from the thought; and the results are the fruits of the action. Just like a seed requires nurturing and caring to grow and develop, you need to transform your thought into action to achieve your goals. By just having profound thoughts and not acting upon them, you create discontent. Getting things done is important because it creates dynamism in your life and every successful action will lead you to perform more such actions effortlessly. We are creatures of habit and by cultivating the habit of doing inspired acts; you are practicing what great men have done. You are awakening the magic that elevates mere action into successful results.

Make a list of the 10 most important things that you need to do in order to transform your life and get the best possible outcomes.

Then go ahead and take inspired action.

"Take time to deliberate but when the time for action arrives, stop thinking and go in." Napoleon Bonaparte

Cause and effect

This universal law is indisputable. Every effect has a cause. Once you recognize and accept this fact, you will realize the importance of taking responsibility for your actions. For example, if someone is overweight, it will eventually lead to sickness and ill health. However, the main cause for someone being overweight is the person himself and his actions. Unless they recognise this fact and take responsibility for their actions, they will not be able to reverse the process and lose weight.

The first step towards being positive is to accept that your own negative and misguided actions led you to the current situation you are in. It takes courage to accept your mistakes but once you do so, it gives you the strength to undo them.

On the other hand, if you refuse to accept your responsibility and find excuses or blame other people or circumstances for being overweight, then you will continue practising unhealthy habits and actions that led you to becoming overweight. This means that you are not willing to change. If you are not willing to change, then how can you expect your situation to change?

Einstein said, "Doing the same thing over and over again and expecting different results is insanity." I say, keep doing things differently until you get the desired outcome. Once you embrace this philosophy, you will not only be able to enrich your life with the immense possibility of getting better results with every inspired action that you perform but you will also be able to awaken and discover the limitless potential that lies untapped within you.

"Shallow men believe in luck or in circumstance. Strong men believe in cause and effect." Ralph Waldo Emerson

Responsibility

If you burn your hands while playing with fire or touching a hot object, then you cannot blame the fire or the hot object for the pain that you experienced. You have to recognize the fact that it was your action – coming in contact with fire or heat – that led to the consequences. This awareness will prevent you from experiencing pain and enable you to take necessary precautions when a similar situation arises in the future.

Responsibility is your ability to respond to the situations in your life and becoming aware of your actions that led you to a particular situation. Most people resist responsibility and thereby become puppets who are the willing victims of their own actions. Once you accept responsibility for your actions, you will realize that achieving your goals is not an uphill task as most people make it out to be.

Everything that you desire and deserve is within your reach. Everything that happens in your life is because of your own actions. What happens around you does not really affect you but your response and how you react is what really affects you. So, if you feel pain or anger, happiness or confidence, it is because your mind has allowed these emotions to be experienced in reaction to what's happening around you. So, focus on controlling your mind and your actions, and when you see the positive change in yourself, you will be able to influence and effect a positive change in the people and the situations around you.

"In dreams begin responsibilities." W. B. Yeats

Stories and examples

I have worked with hundreds of people and witnessed amazing results because these people were willing to take responsibility and improve their situation by making necessary changes in their thinking, in their actions, in the food they eat and in their lifestyle.

I will share an example of a client with whom I worked to demonstrate that you can improve your situation no matter what, if you are willing to make changes and turn away from the path that leads to unhappiness, sickness and ill health and embark upon a new journey towards fitness, good health and happiness.

You can turn around your life by making very simple changes and transform your life for the better.

My client had reached one of the lowest points in life when he contacted me and expressed a desire and willingness to change. We worked on gaining a deeper understanding what had caused the unhealthy and unhappy situation. The important thing was to look beyond superficial symptoms and address the main causes. When I started working with him, more and more issues and challenges came to the surface but I knew that changing yourself from the inside out is similar to the herbal process of healing, you get worse before you start getting better.

In three months, my client was able to gain clarity of his goals and define why they were important in his life, and garner support from family and friends. He took the necessary actions which eventually transformed his life. In 12 weeks, not only did he lose 2 ½ stone but also improved his food choices, his way of thinking, his lifestyle, his self-esteem and his relationships. He was able to take precautions and prevent sickness, and also overcome minor health setbacks easily and effortlessly. The happiness and health that he experienced was felt all around him, among his family members and friends.

This demonstrates that by applying the information and knowledge in this book, combined with a positive attitude and inspired action, an individual can bring about change within and around him. So empower yourself with this newfound knowledge, to embark on a journey towards health and happiness and you will witness that the enthusiasm and excitement you feel within you will start spreading among the people you come into contact with.

"You believe that things or people make you unhappy but this is not accurate. You make yourself unhappy." Wayne Dyer

Chapter 7

Powered transformational change

There's no going back

New thinking and attitude

Think that you have the power to change and you will. In this book, you have seen that there is nothing that the mind cannot achieve if you really and sincerely think it can be done.

Your mind is a blank canvas and your thoughts are the colours with which you paint to create a picture of your life. You are the artist and the creator of your life. Use bright colours or positive thoughts to paint a happy and healthy picture instead of using dark and harsh colours or negative feelings to create a dull and gloomy portrait of your life. Don't let the knowledge that your life is your responsibility scare you. Use this newfound knowledge to turn your life around and steer it towards your goals and your desires.

Your innermost thoughts possess the power to influence your attitude in life. With every inspired action that you take, you are constantly learning and contributing to your knowledge, experience, wisdom and enlightenment.

Maintain humility. It comes with the awareness that there is a wealth of knowledge to be gained and use this awareness to create a change for the better. Regardless of what is going on in the outside world, focus on your attitude and actions, and influence them with your thoughts from within. Take for example, your goal to lose weight stems from your desire to feel more confident, healthier and happier, and in order to achieve this one of the important things you need to do is eat healthy food. But all around, you see people eating cakes and cookies and other kinds of processed and junk food. What do you do? You listen to your innermost thoughts and allow them to drive your actions.

Your attitude towards eating is derived from your resolve to achieve your ideal weight and shape so that you can fit into the ideal clothes that you have already bought as a source of inspiration and confidence that you will achieve what you want.

"I can't change the direction of the wind but I can adjust my sails to always reach my destination." Jimmy Dean

Flab to FAB™ Detoxing and Cleansing

You have learnt in this book the importance of detoxing and cleansing your body and how radically long-term the benefits of this approach is compared to the crash diets or quick-fix weight-loss programmes which may produce instant gratification through short-lived results but do more harm in the longer run.

Once you adopt and cultivate Flab to FAB™ detoxing and cleansing, you will notice the benefits that it bestows on your body. Your whole system from the inside out begins to radiate health and wellbeing. Your internal organs start functioning to their optimum capacity and your tissues and muscles are energized, every cell in your body radiates the freshness and cleanliness of being pure and you will feel less tired and more energetic to do the things you want to do.

I recommend that you practice Flab to FAB™ detoxing and cleansing 2 to 4 times a year. The best way to do this is to join forces with a likeminded partner or join a group environment. This improves accountability and you gain essential guidance and support to keep you on track to consistently maintain health and wellbeing. The main reason why you need to do the Flab to FAB™ detox and cleanse at regular intervals is because your body is constantly being attacked by external elements through the food and water that you consume, the air you breathe, the clothes you wear and the things that you come into contact with in your daily life. Just like we bathe to clean our body, it is important to cleanse our body from the inside and get rid of harmful toxins and contaminants which prevent us from realizing the full potential that our bodies are capable of.

The more attention we pay to keeping our bodies clean and pure from within, the less susceptible we are to external stress and infections. The result is a healthy, happy and disease-free life.

"Take care of your body. It's the only place you have to live." John Rohn

Smarter food choices

You have already gained knowledge through this book about how important nutrition is to maintain good health and how it contributes to maintaining your ideal body shape and weight. Your relationship with the food that you eat is directly related to the shape and the size of your body. It also determines your energy levels to perform physical and mental activities that constitute living a full life.

Your food is the fuel that energizes your body just like the fuel that you fill in your car is what enables it to function properly. If the quality of fuel that you use in your car is not good, then it can damage your car and eventually lead to a complete breakdown. Similarly what you eat affects the health of your body and mind.

Eating junk food or any kind of comfort food is associated with stress and is a reactive response to seek instant gratification or relief from stress that your mind or body experiences. But it is an ineffective and harmful way to deal with stress because by eating junk food or comfort food, you are trying to fill a gaping and growing hole created by stress that can never be filled. You are wilfully harming your body. To effectively cope with stress, use your mind instead of harming your body.

By clarifying your goals and embarking on a journey towards fitness, health and wellbeing, your ability to cope with stressful situations improves and you become aware that eating the wrong food is not the ideal way.

Your attitude and behaviour towards food should be proactive and not reactive. Make the decision to eat smart. Choose what to eat based on your goal of achieving your ideal body shape and weight. This decision is independent of external and temporary influences such as stress or temptation.

One of the most common misconceptions is that healthy food is not tasty and this is a myth or fallacy propagated by lazy thoughts and negative minds. As demonstrated by world famous chefs and cooking experts, by tapping into your creative capacity you can prepare dishes that are not only tasty but also healthy.

Laziness, lack of imagination and a closed and negative mindset is what prevent us from experimenting and trying out new and innovative food preparations. Once you start making smarter food choices, your diet will be enriched with a variety that you never experienced before and you will realize not only the limitations of fast food or comfort food but also how much easier it is to eat healthy.

So make smarter food choices and you will not have to work harder to maintain your health and wellbeing.

"To eat is a necessity but to eat intelligently is an art." Francois de La Rochefoucauld

Effective Exercise

There is no need to work hard and long if you are smart. You have learnt in this book how it is actually possible to achieve more by doing less. You also do not have to force yourself to do the things that you do not want to and can instead do movements that you enjoy. By doing the right kind of movements for just 10 to 40 minutes a day, 3 to 5 times a week, it is possible to improve your metabolism, health and achieve your ideal body shape and weight. To gain a fully functional lean and healthy body, you don't have to forego doing the things you enjoy and spend hours at the gym.

Turn your body from a fat-storing machine to a fat-burning machine without using any kind of expensive xercise equipment. Visit my website www.flabtofabbook.com, and get a programme that is tailored to your requirements. Do less and achieve more.

Isn't this like being offered health on a platter?

It is and the simple reason it is so is because the journey to fitness and health is not at all difficult when you know the way and have the benefit of a knowledgeable guide.

Contrary to what you have been told, you can enjoy the process of getting healthy and fit. That's exactly why I created this holistic health, fitness and wellbeing programme and I am offering it to you on a platter. All you have to do is take it and use it.

"Motivation is what gets you started. Habit is what keeps you going." Jim Ryun

Better view of self

I am not good enough. It's not something I can do. I can't do it. I haven't done anything like this before. It's not possible.

Stop yourself right there when you hear yourself speak like this or even think like this. This is the characteristic of a sick and weak mind. When you hear someone say they can't, what they really mean is they won't. You are deciding that you cannot do something without even trying because you have a negative mindset. Because of their environment, past experiences or through the influence of others, most people have been conditioned to devalue their abilities and potential and feel worthless and hopeless. They enjoy wallowing in self-pity because it is easier to do nothing. When you take positive action you know you cannot expect good things to happen on their own but that you have to make them happen.

A lazy mindset is also a negative mindset.

I strongly believe in my own ability to be healthy and happy. I believe that you deserve to see yourself in the best positive light because your potential is unlimited. Your potential is like the tip of an iceberg and you cannot fathom the greatness that lies within.

From my own experience, I can tell you that I was my own worst enemy because I used to tell myself that I wasn't good enough, putting myself down at every point and by doing so I was giving myself permission to fail. The negativity in my mind had reached such enormous proportions that I didn't know how to deal with it. My mind became a dark and dreary place. I suffered a major setback and was severely ill for over a year. The cause was not external but internal. It was in my mind and only when I realized this could I recover completely. I am telling you this because I do not want you to lose a year suffering from negativity like I did. I applied all that is mentioned in this book to transform my life, achieve health and happiness, and enrich the quality of my life. I returned from a dark and dreary place to reclaim the light and joy that is rightfully mine.

On my website www.flabtofabbook.com, I will show you some simple techniques to immediately turnaround your mind positively, prevent it from wallowing in self-pity, and start valuing the potential you possess to develop and enrich your life.

"A great deal of the chaos in the world occurs because people don't appreciate themselves." Chogyam Trungpa

Your new superstar lifestyle

When other people start seeing you the way you see yourself, you will realize that you are a superstar and the superstar lifestyle that you always wanted is within your reach. Other people will respect and love you only if you respect and love yourself.

This is an indisputable fact.

If you feel that you do not have the respect or the love of others, you have no one to blame but yourself. When you start loving yourself and respecting and recognizing your potential, then the love, respect and confidence from within you will emanate and influence the people around you. You will experience that other people are seeing you in a new light.

Doors and opportunities that hitherto were closed to you suddenly begin to open and welcome you. The superstar lifestyle that you desire and deserve can be yours if you want it to be.

Everyone on this planet is a star whose potential to shine and emit radiance lies hidden until the individual discovers this potential.

It is important to maintain your humility and balance after you have realized your potential so that you don't burn out your superstar radiance and revert to a black hole of negativity. You now know that how you see yourself is how others see you.

The important thing to ask is, what is my true superstar lifestyle? This will bring clarity in your mind about what you desire.

Write down a list of 5 to 10 things that define what your ideal lifestyle entails.

"Your lifestyle – how you live, eat, emote and think – determines your health." Brian Carter

Support Group

You have learnt that you cannot really control people or situations. The only thing you can control is yourself. At the same time, the people around you can have a great influence on your mindset. If you are surrounded by negative people, then it becomes very difficult for you to sustain a positive mindset.

It is therefore important to surround yourself with positive likeminded people and interact with them so that they provide you the necessary support to reach your goals and also hold you accountable for not tapping into your strengths.

Today, with greater awareness and technology, there are many easy ways to seek support and find a group of likeminded people with whom you can share and exchange ideas and encouragement.

Here are 7 steps to get you started in finding the right support to achieve your goals.

1. Join an online group on a social media forum such as Google+ or Facebook. If you want, you can even create an online group and invite others to join you.

2. Join a live or online Mastermind group. A Mastermind group is basically an interactive set of people who are experts in a particular field and enables members to co-ordinate efforts and exchange knowledge in a spirit of harmony.

3. Make a list of people whom you may need to contact, in case you need to clarify something. There is nothing better than talking and discussing things with someone who understands you and whom you can trust and who will hold you accountable.

4. Your support can also come from a source of knowledge such as reading a book or listening to an audio book which will fill your mind with positive and inspiring thoughts.

5. Maintain a log or journal where you can write down your positive statements and thoughts and also keep track of your progress.

6. Confide in your nearest and dearest people. It could be your partner or your immediate family or friends with whom you can share your innermost thoughts.

7. Attend a relevant course or seminar which will enrich your knowledge and guide you in a systematic manner to achieve your goals.

Your journey towards achieving your goals and desires can often be very lonely and the more positive support systems and networks you build around you, the faster and easier it becomes to achieve them.

"When you want something, the universe conspires in helping you to achieve it." Paulo Coelho

Past, Present and Future

Your perspective of your past, present and future is very important and it has a direct impact on your life.

Most people have a tendency to live 80% of their lives based on past experiences, 15% of their lives anticipating or worrying about the future and only 5% of their life is focussed on the here and now. It is a pity because as Master Oogway, the wise turtle in the movie, Kung Fu Panda, says, "Yesterday is history, tomorrow is a mystery, but today is a gift. That is why it is called the present."

Whatever happened in the past, you cannot change. What is going to happen in the future is something you do not know nor can control. What's happening now will eventually become a part of your past and also influence the future. So, doesn't it make sense that you live in the moment and exploit the opportunities that you have right now, right here instead of dwelling on the past or worrying about the future?

Therefore, forget your failures and unsuccessful attempts to lose weight in the past. Use the newfound knowledge that you now possess to move closer towards your goals and most importantly, enjoy the process. If you do something you think and know you will regret later, don't do it. If something makes you feel good then it is a sign that you should continue doing it.

"It is not uncommon for people to spend their whole life waiting to start living." Eckhart Tolle

Putting it all together

Mindset: You are what you think.

Nutrition: You are what you eat.

Exercise: You are how you move.

Lifestyle: You are as great as you want to be.

These are the four fundamental components to achieve a well-balanced, harmonious and inspiring life. They are important to success just the way air is important to breathe, food to satiate hunger, thought is to the mind and mindfulness of action is to effectiveness. The whole is the sum of the parts and one element without the other is ineffectual. All you need to do is think, eat, move, play and be.

How you do it is the question. I hope that you will be able to derive value from this knowledge and apply the learning you have gained from this book and use it in a productive manner to transform and enrich your life.

You are the light. So travel light and let your light shine bright to make this world alight. Use your light to do the things that you think and know are right.

"Think well. Eat right. Do good. Live great. Become the star that you are."
Vishal Morjaria